PCOS COOKBOOK FOR WOMEN

Reclaim Your Health with Delicious and Nutritious PCOS-Friendly Recipes!

By Emily Smith

TABLE OF CONTENTS

Chapter 3: PCOS Diet Dinner Recipes........... 47

Chapter 6: PCOS Diet Beverages Recipes..... 93

INTRODUCTION

Once upon a time, there was a young woman named Sarah who had just been diagnosed with PCOS. At first, she didn't know what it meant or how it would affect her life. But as she learned more about the condition, she realized that it could have serious consequences for her health.

PCOS, or polycystic ovary syndrome, is a hormonal disorder that affects many women. It can cause a range of symptoms, including irregular periods, weight gain, acne, and infertility. But one of the most serious complications of PCOS is insulin resistance, which can lead to diabetes and other health problems.

Sarah was determined not to let PCOS control her life. She wanted to take charge of her health and find a way to manage her symptoms. She knew that diet could play a key role in this, so she began to research the best foods to eat for PCOS.

One of the main dietary recommendations for women with PCOS is to follow a low-glycemic index (GI) diet. This means avoiding foods that cause a rapid spike in blood sugar, such as refined carbohydrates and sugary drinks. Instead, Sarah learned to focus on whole, nutrient-dense foods that would help stabilize her blood sugar and support her overall health.

Some of the best foods for women with PCOS include:

- Non-starchy vegetables, such as leafy greens, broccoli, and cauliflower
- Lean protein sources, such as chicken, fish, and tofu
- Healthy fats, such as olive oil, nuts, and avocado
- Low-glycemic fruits, such as berries and cherries

Sarah found that incorporating these foods into her diet helped her manage her PCOS symptoms more effectively. She felt more energized and less bloated, and her skin began to clear up. She also began to lose weight, which was a welcome bonus.

But Sarah knew that diet alone wasn't enough to manage her PCOS. She also needed to be physically active and manage her stress levels. She started going for regular walks in the park, doing yoga, and practicing mindfulness meditation. These activities helped her feel more relaxed and centered, and they also helped her maintain a healthy weight.

As Sarah continued on her PCOS journey, she discovered that there were many other women out there who were struggling with the same condition. She found a support group online and began sharing her experiences with other women who understood what she was going through. She also became an advocate for PCOS awareness, spreading the word about the condition and encouraging other women to take charge of their health.

Through it all, Sarah learned that managing PCOS was a journey, not a destination. It required patience, perseverance, and a willingness to try new things. But with the right diet, exercise, and self-care, she knew that she could live a healthy, happy life despite her PCOS.

In conclusion, PCOS can have serious consequences for women's health, but it doesn't have to be a life sentence. By following a healthy diet, exercising regularly, and managing stress levels, women with PCOS can manage their symptoms and live a full, vibrant life. It may not be easy, but with determination and support, anything is possible.

Chapter 1: PCOS Diet Breakfast Recipes

Breakfast is often considered the most important meal of the day, and this is especially true for women with PCOS. A healthy breakfast can help regulate blood sugar levels, boost energy, and reduce cravings throughout the day. In this chapter, we'll explore five delicious and nutritious breakfast recipes that are specifically designed for women with PCOS.

Blueberry and Almond Butter Smoothie Bowl

Smoothie bowls are a great way to pack in a variety of nutrients and flavors into one meal. This blueberry and almond butter smoothie bowl is not only delicious but also high in protein and healthy fats.

Ingredients:

- 1 cup frozen blueberries
- 1 ripe banana

- 1/2 cup unsweetened almond milk
- 1/4 cup plain Greek yogurt
- 1 tablespoon almond butter
- 1 teaspoon honey
- 1/4 cup granola
- 1 tablespoon chia seeds
- 1 tablespoon sliced almonds

Instructions:

1. In a blender, combine the frozen blueberries, banana, almond milk, Greek yogurt, almond butter, and honey. Blend until smooth and creamy.
2. Pour the smoothie into a bowl and top with granola, chia seeds, and sliced almonds.
3. Enjoy immediately.

Vegetable and Egg White Frittata

This vegetable and egg white frittata is a great way to get in a serving of veggies first thing in the morning. Plus, it's high in protein and low in carbs.

Ingredients:

- 1 tablespoon olive oil
- 1/2 red onion, diced
- 1 bell pepper, diced
- 1 zucchini, diced
- 6 egg whites
- 2 whole eggs
- 1/4 cup grated Parmesan cheese
- Salt and pepper, to taste

Instructions:

1. Preheat the oven to 350°F.
2. Heat the olive oil in a 10-inch oven-safe skillet over medium heat. Add the onion, bell pepper, and zucchini and cook until the vegetables are tender, about 5 minutes.
3. In a separate bowl, whisk together the egg whites, whole eggs, Parmesan cheese, salt, and pepper.

4. Pour the egg mixture over the vegetables in the skillet and cook for 2-3 minutes, until the edges start to set.

5. Transfer the skillet to the oven and bake for 10-15 minutes, until the frittata is set and golden brown on top.

6. Slice and serve hot.

Low-Carb Zucchini and Bacon Breakfast Casserole

This low-carb breakfast casserole is packed with protein and healthy fats, thanks to the bacon and eggs. Plus, it's a great way to use up any extra zucchini you may have in your fridge.

Ingredients:

- 1 tablespoon olive oil
- 2 zucchini, sliced
- 6 slices bacon, cooked and crumbled
- 8 eggs
- 1/2 cup heavy cream

- 1/2 cup shredded cheddar cheese
- Salt and pepper, to taste

Instructions:

1. Preheat the oven to 375°F.
2. Heat the olive oil in a large skillet over medium-high heat. Add the zucchini and cook until tender, about 5 minutes.
3. In a separate bowl, whisk together the eggs, heavy cream, shredded cheddar cheese, salt, and pepper.
4. Grease a 9x13 inch baking dish and add the cooked zucchini to the bottom of the dish. Pour the egg mixture over the zucchini and top with the crumbled bacon.
5. Bake for 25-30 minutes, until the casserole is set and the top is golden brown.
6. Let cool for a few minutes before slicing and serving.

Cinnamon and Vanilla Chia Pudding

Chia seeds are a great source of fiber, protein, and omega-3 fatty acids. This cinnamon and vanilla chia pudding is a delicious and nutritious way to start your day.

Ingredients:

- 1/4 cup chia seeds
- 1 cup unsweetened almond milk
- 1 tablespoon honey
- 1 teaspoon vanilla extract
- 1/2 teaspoon ground cinnamon

Instructions:

1. In a medium bowl, whisk together the chia seeds, almond milk, honey, vanilla extract, and ground cinnamon.
2. Cover the bowl and refrigerate for at least 2 hours, or overnight, until the chia seeds have absorbed the liquid and the mixture has thickened.

3. Stir the pudding before serving and top with fresh berries or sliced almonds.

Oatmeal and Banana Protein Pancakes

These oatmeal and banana protein pancakes are a healthy and delicious twist on traditional pancakes. They're high in protein and fiber, making them a great breakfast option for women with PCOS.

Ingredients:

- 1 ripe banana, mashed
- 2 eggs
- 1/2 cup rolled oats
- 1/2 scoop vanilla protein powder
- 1/2 teaspoon ground cinnamon
- 1/4 teaspoon baking powder
- 1/4 cup unsweetened almond milk

Instructions:

1. In a medium bowl, whisk together the mashed banana, eggs, rolled oats, vanilla protein powder, ground cinnamon, baking powder, and unsweetened almond milk.
2. Heat a nonstick skillet over medium heat and lightly coat with cooking spray.
3. Pour 1/4 cup of the pancake batter onto the skillet and cook until the edges start to set and the bottom is golden brown, about 2-3 minutes.
4. Flip the pancake and cook for an additional 1-2 minutes on the other side.
5. Repeat with the remaining pancake batter, making sure to lightly coat the skillet with cooking spray between each pancake.
6. Serve hot with fresh fruit or a drizzle of honey.

Sweet Potato Breakfast Bowl

This sweet potato breakfast bowl is a hearty and filling breakfast that's packed with fiber, protein, and healthy fats.

Ingredients:

- 1 medium sweet potato, peeled and diced
- 1 tablespoon olive oil
- 1/2 teaspoon smoked paprika
- 1/2 teaspoon garlic powder
- 1/4 teaspoon sea salt
- 2 large eggs
- 1/2 avocado, sliced
- 2 tablespoons chopped fresh cilantro
- 1/4 lime, juiced

Instructions:

1. Preheat the oven to 400°F (200°C).
2. Toss the diced sweet potato with the olive oil, smoked paprika, garlic powder, and sea salt. Spread out on a baking sheet and roast for 20-25 minutes, until tender and lightly browned.
3. In a small skillet, cook the eggs to your preference.

4. Divide the roasted sweet potato between two bowls. Top each with a cooked egg, avocado slices, chopped cilantro, and a squeeze of lime juice.

Berry and Coconut Yogurt Parfait

This berry and coconut yogurt parfait is a refreshing and satisfying breakfast that's loaded with antioxidants, fiber, and healthy fats.

Ingredients:

- 1 cup plain Greek yogurt
- 1/2 cup fresh or frozen mixed berries
- 1/4 cup unsweetened shredded coconut
- 1 tablespoon honey
- 1/4 teaspoon vanilla extract

Instructions:

1. In a small bowl, mix together the Greek yogurt, honey, and vanilla extract.

2. In a separate bowl, gently toss the mixed berries with the shredded coconut.

3. To assemble the parfait, spoon a layer of the yogurt mixture into the bottom of a glass or jar. Top with a layer of the berry and coconut mixture. Repeat until all ingredients are used up.

4. Serve immediately or cover and refrigerate for later.

Almond Butter and Banana Smoothie

This almond butter and banana smoothie is a quick and easy breakfast that's high in protein, fiber, and healthy fats.

Ingredients:

- 1 ripe banana
- 1 tablespoon almond butter
- 1/2 cup unsweetened almond milk
- 1/2 scoop vanilla protein powder
- 1/2 teaspoon ground cinnamon
- 1/4 teaspoon vanilla extract
- 1 cup ice cubes

Instructions:

1. In a blender, combine the banana, almond butter, almond milk, vanilla protein powder, ground cinnamon, vanilla extract, and ice cubes.
2. Blend until smooth and creamy.
3. Pour into a glass and enjoy immediately.

Vegetable Frittata

This vegetable frittata is a savory and satisfying breakfast that's loaded with protein, fiber, and antioxidants.

Ingredients:

1. 1 tablespoon olive oil
2. 1/2 cup diced bell peppers
3. 1/2 cup diced zucchini
4. 1/2 cup chopped kale
5. 1/4 teaspoon sea salt
6. 4 large eggs
7. 1/4 cup unsweetened almond milk
8. 1/4 teaspoon black pepper

9. 1/4 teaspoon dried oregano

Instructions:

1. Preheat the oven to 350°F (175°C).
2. In a 10-inch oven-safe skillet, heat the olive oil over medium heat. Add the bell peppers, zucchini, kale, and sea salt. Cook for 5-7 minutes, until the vegetables are tender and lightly browned.
3. In a medium bowl, whisk together the eggs, almond milk, black pepper, and dried oregano.

Starting your day with a healthy breakfast is essential for women with PCOS. These five delicious and nutritious breakfast recipes are packed with protein, healthy fats, and fiber, and are specifically designed to help regulate blood sugar levels and reduce cravings throughout the day. So why not try one of these recipes tomorrow morning and start your day off right!

Chapter 2: PCOS Diet Lunch Recipes

Lunch is an important meal of the day as it helps refuel the body and brain with energy after a long morning. For women with PCOS, it's crucial to choose foods that help stabilize blood sugar levels and reduce inflammation in the body. In this chapter, we'll explore 10 delicious and nutritious lunch recipes that are easy to prepare and perfect for women with PCOS.

Asian-inspired Tuna Salad Lettuce Wraps

Ingredients:

- 2 cans of tuna, drained
- 1/4 cup of mayonnaise
- 1 tablespoon of soy sauce
- 1 teaspoon of honey
- 1 teaspoon of rice vinegar
- 1 teaspoon of sesame oil
- 1/2 teaspoon of grated ginger

- 1/4 teaspoon of red pepper flakes
- 4 large lettuce leaves

Instructions:

1. In a medium bowl, mix together the tuna, mayonnaise, soy sauce, honey, rice vinegar, sesame oil, ginger, and red pepper flakes.
2. Spoon the tuna mixture onto each lettuce leaf and wrap it up tightly.
3. Serve immediately and enjoy.

Chickpea and Sweet Potato Buddha Bowl

Ingredients:

- 1 sweet potato, peeled and chopped
- 1 can of chickpeas, drained and rinsed
- 1/2 red onion, sliced
- 1 red bell pepper, sliced
- 1 tablespoon of olive oil
- 1/2 teaspoon of paprika

- 1/2 teaspoon of cumin
- Salt and pepper to taste
- 2 cups of cooked quinoa
- 1/4 cup of hummus
- 1/4 cup of chopped fresh parsley

Instructions:

1. Preheat the oven to 400°F.
2. In a large bowl, mix together the sweet potato, chickpeas, red onion, red bell pepper, olive oil, paprika, cumin, salt, and pepper.
3. Spread the mixture onto a baking sheet and roast in the oven for 20-25 minutes, or until the sweet potato is tender.
4. To assemble the Buddha bowl, divide the cooked quinoa between two bowls and top with the roasted vegetables.
5. Add a dollop of hummus on top of the vegetables and sprinkle with chopped parsley.
6. Serve immediately and enjoy.

Italian-style Chicken and Vegetable Skewers

Ingredients:

- 2 boneless, skinless chicken breasts, cut into chunks
- 1 zucchini, sliced
- 1 yellow squash, sliced
- 1 red onion, sliced
- 1 red bell pepper, sliced
- 2 tablespoons of olive oil
- 1 tablespoon of dried Italian seasoning
- Salt and pepper to taste

Instructions:

1. Preheat a grill or grill pan to medium-high heat.
2. Thread the chicken and vegetables onto skewers.
3. In a small bowl, whisk together the olive oil, Italian seasoning, salt, and pepper.
4. Brush the skewers with the oil mixture.
5. Grill the skewers for 10-12 minutes, or until the chicken is cooked through.

6.   Serve immediately and enjoy.

Creamy Broccoli and Cauliflower Soup

Ingredients:

- 1 tablespoon of olive oil
- 1 onion, chopped
- 3 garlic cloves, minced
- 4 cups of chicken or vegetable broth
- 1 head of broccoli, chopped
- 1 head of cauliflower, chopped
- 1/2 cup of heavy cream
- Salt and pepper to taste

Instructions:

1.   In a large pot, heat the olive oil over medium heat.
2.   Add the chopped onion and garlic to the pot and sauté until the onion is translucent.
3.   Add the chicken or vegetable broth to the pot and bring it to a boil.

4. Add the chopped broccoli and cauliflower to the pot and simmer for 15-20 minutes, or until the vegetables are tender.

5. Use an immersion blender or transfer the soup to a blender to puree until smooth.

6. Stir in the heavy cream and season with salt and pepper to taste.

7. Serve immediately and enjoy.

Turkey and Avocado Wrap

Ingredients:

- 1 whole wheat tortilla
- 2 slices of turkey breast
- 1/4 avocado, sliced
- 1/4 cup of spinach leaves
- 1/4 cup of shredded carrots
- 1 tablespoon of hummus

Instructions:

1. Lay the tortilla flat on a clean surface.

2. Spread the hummus on the tortilla, leaving a 1-inch border around the edges.

3. Layer the turkey slices, avocado, spinach leaves, and shredded carrots on top of the hummus.

4. Roll up the tortilla tightly, tucking in the sides as you go.

5. Cut the wrap in half and serve immediately.

Greek Salad with Grilled Chicken

Ingredients:

- 2 boneless, skinless chicken breasts
- 1 head of romaine lettuce, chopped
- 1/2 cup of cherry tomatoes, halved
- 1/2 cup of sliced cucumber
- 1/4 cup of sliced red onion
- 1/4 cup of crumbled feta cheese
- 1 tablespoon of red wine vinegar
- 2 tablespoons of olive oil
- Salt and pepper to taste

Instructions:

1. Preheat a grill or grill pan to medium-high heat.

2. Season the chicken breasts with salt and pepper.

3. Grill the chicken breasts for 6-8 minutes per side, or until cooked through.

4. In a large bowl, combine the chopped romaine lettuce, cherry tomatoes, sliced cucumber, sliced red onion, and crumbled feta cheese.

5. In a small bowl, whisk together the red wine vinegar, olive oil, salt, and pepper.

6. Toss the salad with the dressing and divide it between two plates.

7. Top each salad with a grilled chicken breast.

8. Serve immediately and enjoy.

Spaghetti Squash Pad Thai

Ingredients:

- 1 spaghetti squash, halved and seeded
- 2 tablespoons of olive oil
- 1 onion, chopped

- 2 garlic cloves, minced
- 2 carrots, peeled and julienned
- 2 red bell peppers, julienned
- 1/4 cup of peanut butter
- 2 tablespoons of soy sauce
- 1 tablespoon of honey
- 1 tablespoon of lime juice
- 1/4 teaspoon of red pepper flakes
- 1/4 cup of chopped fresh cilantro
- 1/4 cup of chopped peanuts

Instructions:

1. Preheat the oven to 375°F.
2. Brush the cut sides of the spaghetti squash with olive oil and place them cut-side down on a baking sheet.
3. Bake the spaghetti squash for 35-40 minutes, or until tender.
4. In a large skillet, heat the olive oil over medium-high heat.
5. Add the onion and garlic to the skillet and sauté until the onion is translucent.

6. Add the julienned carrots and red bell peppers to the skillet and sauté until the vegetables are tender.

7. In a small bowl, whisk together the peanut butter, soy sauce, honey, lime juice, and red pepper flakes.

8. Use a fork to scrape the spaghetti squash flesh into the skillet with the vegetables.

9. Pour the peanut butter sauce over the spaghetti squash and vegetables and stir to combine.

10. Cook for an additional 2-3 minutes, or until heated through.

11. Divide the pad thai between two plates and top with chopped cilantro and chopped peanuts.

12. Serve immediately and enjoy.

Black Bean and Sweet Potato Quesadillas

Ingredients:

- 1 large sweet potato, peeled and diced
- 1 tablespoon of olive oil
- 1/2 teaspoon of chili powder
- Salt and pepper to taste

- 4 whole wheat tortillas

- 1 can of black beans, drained and rinsed

- 1/2 cup of shredded cheddar cheese

- 1 avocado, sliced

- Salsa and sour cream for serving

Instructions:

1. Preheat the oven to 375°F.

2. Toss the diced sweet potato with olive oil, chili powder, salt, and pepper.

3. Spread the sweet potato in an even layer on a baking sheet and roast for 25-30 minutes, or until tender.

4. Lay the tortillas flat on a clean surface.

5. Divide the roasted sweet potato, black beans, and shredded cheddar cheese evenly among the tortillas, placing the ingredients on one half of each tortilla.

6. Fold the other half of each tortilla over the filling to create a half-moon shape.

7. Heat a large skillet over medium-high heat.

8. Cook the quesadillas for 2-3 minutes per side, or until the tortillas are golden brown and the cheese is melted.

9. Cut each quesadilla into wedges and serve with sliced avocado, salsa, and sour cream.

Grilled Chicken and Veggie Kabobs

Ingredients:

- 2 boneless, skinless chicken breasts, cut into cubes
- 1 red bell pepper, cut into 1-inch pieces
- 1 yellow bell pepper, cut into 1-inch pieces
- 1 zucchini, sliced
- 1 yellow squash, sliced
- 1/2 red onion, cut into wedges
- 1/4 cup of olive oil
- 2 tablespoons of balsamic vinegar
- 2 garlic cloves, minced
- 1 teaspoon of dried oregano
- Salt and pepper to taste

Instructions:

1. Preheat a grill or grill pan to medium-high heat.
2. Thread the chicken cubes, bell pepper pieces, zucchini slices, yellow squash slices, and red onion wedges onto skewers.
3. In a small bowl, whisk together the olive oil, balsamic vinegar, minced garlic, dried oregano, salt, and pepper.
4. Brush the kabobs with the olive oil mixture.
5. Grill the kabobs for 10-12 minutes, turning occasionally, or until the chicken is cooked through and the vegetables are tender.
6. Serve immediately and enjoy.

Tuna Salad Lettuce Wraps

Ingredients:

- 2 cans of tuna, drained
- 1/4 cup of mayonnaise
- 2 tablespoons of Dijon mustard
- 1 tablespoon of lemon juice

- Salt and pepper to taste
- 8 large lettuce leaves
- 1/2 cup of cherry tomatoes, halved
- 1/4 cup of sliced red onion

Instructions:

1. In a medium bowl, combine the drained tuna, mayonnaise, Dijon mustard, lemon juice, salt, and pepper.
2. Mix until well combined.
3. Lay out the lettuce leaves on a clean surface.
4. Divide the tuna salad evenly among the lettuce leaves, placing the tuna mixture in the center of each leaf.
5. Top the tuna salad with cherry tomato halves and sliced red onion.
6. Roll up the lettuce leaves around the tuna salad, securing with toothpicks if needed.
7. Serve immediately and enjoy.

Chickpea and Vegetable Buddha Bowl

Ingredients:

- 1 cup of cooked quinoa
- 1 can of chickpeas, drained and rinsed
- 1 zucchini, sliced
- 1 yellow squash, sliced
- 1 red bell pepper, sliced
- 1 tablespoon of olive oil
- 1 teaspoon of smoked paprika
- Salt and pepper to taste
- 2 cups of spinach
- 1 avocado, sliced
- Lemon wedges for serving

Instructions:

1. Preheat the oven to 400°F.
2. Toss the sliced zucchini, yellow squash, and red bell pepper with olive oil, smoked paprika, salt, and pepper.

3. Spread the vegetables in an even layer on a baking sheet and roast for 25-30 minutes, or until tender and lightly charred.

4. Assemble the buddha bowls by dividing the cooked quinoa, chickpeas, roasted vegetables, spinach, and sliced avocado between two bowls.

5. Serve with lemon wedges on the side.

Turkey and Veggie Wrap

Ingredients:

- 2 whole wheat tortillas
- 4 ounces of deli turkey
- 1/2 cup of shredded carrots
- 1/2 cup of sliced cucumber
- 1/4 cup of hummus
- 1/4 cup of crumbled feta cheese

Instructions:

1. Lay the tortillas flat on a clean surface.

2. Divide the deli turkey, shredded carrots, sliced cucumber, hummus, and crumbled feta cheese evenly between the tortillas, placing the ingredients in the center of each tortilla.

3. Fold the sides of each tortilla inwards and then roll up the tortilla tightly to create a wrap.

4. Slice the wraps in half and serve immediately.

Italian Chopped Salad

Ingredients:

- 4 cups of chopped romaine lettuce
- 1 cup of chopped radicchio
- 1 cup of chopped endive
- 1 cup of chopped cherry tomatoes
- 1/2 cup of chopped salami
- 1/2 cup of chopped provolone cheese
- 1/4 cup of chopped red onion
- 1/4 cup of chopped fresh parsley
- 1/4 cup of chopped fresh basil
- 1/4 cup of olive oil
- 2 tablespoons of red wine vinegar

- 1 teaspoon of Dijon mustard
- Salt and pepper to taste

Instructions:

1. In a large bowl, combine the chopped romaine lettuce, radicchio, endive, cherry tomatoes, salami, provolone cheese, red onion, parsley, and basil.
2. In a small bowl, whisk together the olive oil, red wine vinegar, Dijon mustard, salt, and pepper.
3. Pour the dressing over the salad and toss to combine.
4. Divide the salad between two plates and serve immediately.

Vegan Lentil Soup

Ingredients:

- 1 tablespoon of olive oil
- 1 onion, chopped
- 2 carrots, peeled and chopped
- 2 celery stalks, chopped
- 3 garlic cloves, minced

- 1 teaspoon of ground cumin
- 1/2 teaspoon of smoked paprika
- 1/2 teaspoon of dried thyme
- 1/2 teaspoon of dried oregano
- Salt and pepper to taste
- 1 cup of red lentils
- 4 cups of vegetable broth
- 1 can of diced tomatoes, undrained
- 1/2 cups of chopped kale
- 1 lemon, juiced
- Fresh parsley for garnish

Instructions:

1. Heat the olive oil in a large pot over medium heat.
2. Add the chopped onion, carrots, celery, and garlic to the pot and sauté for 5-7 minutes, or until the vegetables are tender.
3. Add the ground cumin, smoked paprika, dried thyme, dried oregano, salt, and pepper to the pot and stir to combine.

4. Add the red lentils, vegetable broth, and diced tomatoes to the pot and bring to a boil.

5. Reduce the heat to low and simmer for 25-30 minutes, or until the lentils are tender.

6. Stir in the chopped kale and lemon juice and simmer for an additional 5 minutes.

7. Divide the soup between two bowls and garnish with fresh parsley.

Tofu and Vegetable Stir-Fry

Ingredients:

- 1 tablespoon of vegetable oil
- 1 block of extra-firm tofu, drained and pressed
- 1 red bell pepper, sliced
- 1 yellow bell pepper, sliced
- 1 zucchini, sliced
- 1/2 cup of sliced mushrooms
- 2 garlic cloves, minced
- 1 tablespoon of soy sauce
- 1 tablespoon of hoisin sauce
- 1/4 cup of chopped green onions

- Sesame seeds for garnish

Instructions:

1. Heat the vegetable oil in a large skillet or wok over high heat.
2. Cut the pressed tofu into bite-sized cubes and add them to the hot pan. Stir-fry for 5-7 minutes, or until the tofu is lightly browned on all sides.
3. Add the sliced bell peppers, sliced zucchini, sliced mushrooms, and minced garlic to the pan and stir-fry for an additional 5-7 minutes, or until the vegetables are tender-crisp.
4. In a small bowl, whisk together the soy sauce and hoisin sauce.
5. Add the sauce to the pan and stir to coat the tofu and vegetables evenly.
6. Sprinkle the chopped green onions and sesame seeds over the top of the stir-fry and serve immediately.

Lunchtime can be a challenging meal to plan for when you're looking to eat healthy and stay on track with your goals. But with these ten delicious and nutritious recipes, you'll never be at a loss for lunchtime inspiration. From filling salads and wraps to hearty soups and stews, there's something here for everyone. And with the detailed ingredient lists and step-by-step instructions provided, these recipes are easy to make even if you're not an experienced cook. So go ahead and try them out - your taste buds (and your body) will thank you!

Chapter 3: PCOS Diet Dinner Recipes

Dinner is often the largest meal of the day, and it's important to make sure it's a healthy one. For women with PCOS, dinner can be an opportunity to load up on lean proteins, healthy fats, and fiber-rich vegetables to help manage blood sugar and hormone levels. In this chapter, we'll share 10 delicious and PCOS-friendly dinner recipes that will satisfy your taste buds and nourish your body.

Lemon and Herb Baked Salmon with Asparagus

Ingredients:

- 4 salmon fillets
- 1 bunch of asparagus
- 2 tablespoons of olive oil
- 2 tablespoons of fresh lemon juice
- 1 tablespoon of chopped fresh parsley
- 1 tablespoon of chopped fresh thyme

- 2 cloves of garlic, minced
- Salt and pepper to taste

Instructions:

1. Preheat the oven to 400°F.
2. Rinse the salmon fillets and pat them dry with a paper towel. Season them with salt and pepper and place them in a baking dish.
3. Rinse the asparagus and trim the ends. Arrange them around the salmon fillets in the baking dish.
4. In a small bowl, whisk together the olive oil, lemon juice, parsley, thyme, garlic, salt, and pepper.
5. Pour the mixture over the salmon and asparagus, making sure to coat everything evenly.
6. Bake in the oven for 12-15 minutes, or until the salmon is cooked through and the asparagus is tender.
7. Serve hot and enjoy!

Moroccan-style Chickpea and Vegetable Stew

Ingredients:

- 1 tablespoon of olive oil
- 1 large onion, chopped
- 3 garlic cloves, minced
- 2 teaspoons of ground cumin
- 1 teaspoon of ground cinnamon
- 1 teaspoon of ground coriander
- 1/4 teaspoon of cayenne pepper
- 2 cups of vegetable broth
- 2 cups of canned chickpeas, drained and rinsed
- 2 cups of diced tomatoes
- 2 cups of diced butternut squash
- 1 cup of diced carrot
- 1 cup of diced celery
- Salt and pepper to taste
- Fresh cilantro for garnish

Instructions:

1. Heat the olive oil in a large pot over medium heat. Add the onion and garlic and cook until the onion is soft and translucent, about 5 minutes.

2. Add the cumin, cinnamon, coriander, and cayenne pepper and stir to combine. Cook for another 2-3 minutes, or until fragrant.

3. Add the vegetable broth, chickpeas, tomatoes, butternut squash, carrot, and celery. Stir to combine.

4. Bring the mixture to a simmer and then reduce the heat to low. Cover the pot and let the stew cook for 30-40 minutes, or until the vegetables are tender and the flavors have melded together.

5. Season with salt and pepper to taste.

6. Serve hot, garnished with fresh cilantro.

Greek-style Chicken and Vegetable Skillet

Ingredients:

- 4 boneless, skinless chicken breasts, cubed
- 1 red onion, sliced
- 1 red bell pepper, sliced
- 1 yellow bell pepper, sliced
- 2 cups of sliced zucchini
- 1 cup of cherry tomatoes
- 1/4 cup of olive oil
- 2 tablespoons of red wine vinegar
- 2 cloves of garlic, minced
- 1 tablespoon of dried oregano
- Salt and pepper to taste
- Feta cheese for garnish

Instructions:

1. Heat the olive oil in a large skillet over medium-high heat.

2. Add the chicken cubes to the skillet and cook until browned on all sides, about 5-7 minutes.

3. Remove the chicken from the skillet and set it aside on a plate.

4. Add the onion, bell peppers, zucchini, cherry tomatoes, garlic, oregano, salt, and pepper to the skillet.

5. Stir to combine and cook until the vegetables are tender, about 8-10 minutes.

6. Return the chicken to the skillet and add the red wine vinegar.

7. Cook for another 2-3 minutes, or until the chicken is heated through and the flavors have melded together.

8. Serve hot, garnished with crumbled feta cheese.

Spicy Shrimp and Vegetable Stir Fry

Ingredients:

- 1 pound of shrimp, peeled and deveined
- 1 red onion, sliced
- 1 red bell pepper, sliced
- 1 yellow bell pepper, sliced

- 2 cups of sliced broccoli

- 1 cup of sliced snow peas

- 2 tablespoons of olive oil

- 2 tablespoons of soy sauce

- 1 tablespoon of honey

- 1 tablespoon of sriracha

- 2 cloves of garlic, minced

- Salt and pepper to taste

Instructions:

1. Heat the olive oil in a large skillet over medium-high heat.

2. Add the shrimp to the skillet and cook until pink and cooked through, about 2-3 minutes per side.

3. Remove the shrimp from the skillet and set it aside on a plate.

4. Add the onion, bell peppers, broccoli, snow peas, garlic, salt, and pepper to the skillet.

5. Stir to combine and cook until the vegetables are tender, about 8-10 minutes.

6. In a small bowl, whisk together the soy sauce, honey, and sriracha.

7. Pour the mixture over the vegetables and stir to combine.

8. Add the shrimp back to the skillet and stir to combine.

9. Cook for another 2-3 minutes, or until everything is heated through and the flavors have melded together.

10. Serve hot and enjoy!

Grilled Sirloin Steak with Garlic Butter and Roasted Vegetables

Ingredients:

- 4 sirloin steaks
- 1 bunch of asparagus
- 2 red bell peppers, sliced
- 1 yellow bell pepper, sliced
- 2 cups of sliced mushrooms
- 1/4 cup of olive oil
- 2 cloves of garlic, minced
- 1 tablespoon of chopped fresh thyme

- Salt and pepper to taste
- 1/2 cup of butter, softened

Instructions:

1. Preheat the grill to medium-high heat.
2. Rinse the sirloin steaks and pat them dry with a paper towel. Season them with salt and pepper.
3. In a small bowl, whisk together the olive oil, garlic, thyme, salt, and pepper.
4. Brush the mixture over the asparagus, bell peppers, and mushrooms.
5. Grill the sirloin steaks for 3-4 minutes per side, or until cooked to your liking.
6. Remove the steaks from the grill and let them rest for a few minutes.
7. While the steaks are resting, melt the butter in a small saucepan over low heat.
8. Add the minced garlic to the butter and stir to combine.
9. Place the grilled vegetables on a serving platter.
10. Slice the steak and arrange it on top of the vegetables.

11. Drizzle the garlic butter over the steak and vegetables.

12. Serve hot and enjoy your delicious and nutritious grilled sirloin steak with garlic butter and roasted vegetables.

Vegetarian Stuffed Peppers

Ingredients:

- 4 large bell peppers, any color
- 1 cup of cooked quinoa
- 1 cup of black beans, drained and rinsed
- 1 cup of corn kernels
- 1/2 cup of chopped onion
- 2 cloves of garlic, minced
- 1 teaspoon of ground cumin
- 1 teaspoon of chili powder
- 1/2 teaspoon of paprika
- Salt and pepper to taste
- 1/2 cup of shredded cheddar cheese

Instructions:

1. Preheat the oven to 375°F (190°C).
2. Cut off the tops of the bell peppers and remove the seeds and membranes.
3. In a large bowl, mix together the quinoa, black beans, corn, onion, garlic, cumin, chili powder, paprika, salt, and pepper.
4. Stuff the mixture into the bell peppers, packing it in tightly.
5. Place the stuffed peppers in a baking dish and cover with foil.
6. Bake in the preheated oven for 45 minutes.
7. Remove the foil and sprinkle the shredded cheddar cheese over the top of each pepper.
8. Return the peppers to the oven and bake for an additional 10-15 minutes, or until the cheese is melted and bubbly.
9. Remove the peppers from the oven and let them cool for a few minutes.
10. Serve hot and enjoy your delicious and healthy vegetarian stuffed peppers.

Baked Salmon with Lemon and Dill

Ingredients:

- 4 salmon fillets
- 2 tablespoons of olive oil
- 1 tablespoon of lemon juice
- 1 tablespoon of chopped fresh dill
- Salt and pepper to taste

Instructions:

1. Preheat the oven to 400°F (200°C).
2. Rinse the salmon fillets and pat them dry with a paper towel. Season them with salt and pepper.
3. In a small bowl, whisk together the olive oil, lemon juice, and dill.
4. Brush the mixture over the salmon fillets.
5. Place the salmon fillets in a baking dish and bake in the preheated oven for 12-15 minutes, or until the salmon is cooked through and flakes easily with a fork.

6. Remove the salmon from the oven and let it cool for a few minutes.

7. Serve hot and enjoy your delicious and healthy baked salmon with lemon and dill.

Shrimp Scampi Linguine

Ingredients:

- 1 pound of linguine
- 1 pound of shrimp, peeled and deveined
- 1/2 cup of butter
- 2 tablespoons of olive oil
- 4 cloves of garlic, minced
- 1/2 cup of white wine
- 1 tablespoon of lemon juice
- 1/2 teaspoon of red pepper flakes
- Salt and pepper to taste
- 1/4 cup of chopped fresh parsley

Instructions:

1. Cook the linguine according to the package instructions until al dente.

2. Rinse the shrimp and pat them dry with a paper towel. Season them with salt and pepper.

3. In a large skillet, melt the butter and olive oil over medium-high heat.

4. Add the garlic and red pepper flakes to the skillet and sauté for 1-2 minutes, or until fragrant.

5. Add the shrimp to the skillet and cook for 2-3 minutes per side, or until pink and cooked through.

6. Remove the shrimp from the skillet and set it aside on a plate.

7. Add the white wine and lemon juice to the skillet and bring it to a simmer.

8. Add the cooked linguine to the skillet and toss it with the sauce until it is well coated.

9. Add the cooked shrimp back to the skillet and toss it with the linguine and sauce.

10. Sprinkle the chopped parsley over the top of the linguine and shrimp.

11. Serve hot and enjoy your delicious and flavorful shrimp scampi linguine.

Baked Chicken Parmesan

Ingredients:

- 4 boneless, skinless chicken breasts
- 1 cup of seasoned breadcrumbs
- 1/2 cup of grated Parmesan cheese
- 1/2 teaspoon of garlic powder
- Salt and pepper to taste
- 2 eggs, beaten
- 1 cup of marinara sauce
- 1 cup of shredded mozzarella cheese
- Chopped fresh parsley for garnish

Instructions:

1. Preheat the oven to 375°F (190°C).
2. Season the chicken breasts with salt and pepper.
3. In a shallow dish, mix together the breadcrumbs, Parmesan cheese, garlic powder, salt, and pepper.

4. In another shallow dish, beat the eggs.

5. Dip each chicken breast in the beaten eggs and then coat it in the breadcrumb mixture.

6. Place the chicken breasts in a baking dish and bake in the preheated oven for 25-30 minutes, or until the chicken is cooked through and the coating is golden brown.

7. Remove the chicken from the oven and spoon the marinara sauce over the top of each chicken breast.

8. Sprinkle the shredded mozzarella cheese over the top of the marinara sauce.

9. Return the chicken to the oven and bake for an additional 10-15 minutes, or until the cheese is melted and bubbly.

10. Remove the chicken from the oven and let it cool for a few minutes.

11. Sprinkle the chopped parsley over the top of the chicken breasts.

12. Serve hot and enjoy your delicious and comforting baked chicken parmesan.

Chapter 4: PCOS Diet Snacks and Appetizers Recipes

Snacks and appetizers are an important part of any meal, whether you are hosting a party or just looking for something to munch on during the day. This chapter will focus on creating delicious and healthy snacks and appetizers that are perfect for those with PCOS. These recipes are easy to make and are filled with ingredients that are beneficial for those with PCOS, such as nuts, vegetables, and low-sugar fruits.

Spicy Roasted Chickpeas

Chickpeas are a great source of protein and fiber, making them the perfect snack for those with PCOS. This recipe takes roasted chickpeas to the next level by adding a spicy kick.

Ingredients:

- 1 can chickpeas, drained and rinsed
- 1 tbsp olive oil

- 1 tsp smoked paprika
- 1/2 tsp cumin
- 1/4 tsp cayenne pepper
- Salt to taste

Instructions:

1. Preheat your oven to 400°F (200°C).
2. Rinse and drain the chickpeas and pat them dry with a paper towel.
3. In a small bowl, mix together the olive oil, smoked paprika, cumin, cayenne pepper, and salt.
4. Add the chickpeas to the bowl and toss to coat.
5. Spread the chickpeas in a single layer on a baking sheet and roast for 25-30 minutes, or until crispy.
6. Let the chickpeas cool for a few minutes before serving.

Guacamole with Veggie Dippers

Guacamole is a classic snack that is perfect for any occasion. This recipe is made with fresh ingredients and is served with a variety of colorful vegetables, making it a healthy and tasty snack.

Ingredients:

- 2 ripe avocados
- 1/2 red onion, finely chopped
- 1 small tomato, diced
- 1 garlic clove, minced
- 1 lime, juiced
- Salt and pepper to taste
- Assorted vegetables for dipping (carrots, celery, bell peppers, etc.)

Instructions:

1. Cut the avocados in half and remove the pit.
2. Scoop the avocado flesh into a medium bowl and mash with a fork.
3. Add the chopped red onion, diced tomato, minced garlic, and lime juice to the bowl and mix well.
4. Season with salt and pepper to taste.

5. Serve the guacamole with a variety of colorful vegetables for dipping.

Greek-style Yogurt Dip with Whole-grain Pita Chips

This creamy dip is made with Greek-style yogurt and is flavored with garlic, lemon, and fresh herbs. The whole-grain pita chips are the perfect accompaniment, making this a healthy and satisfying snack.

Ingredients:

- 1 cup Greek-style yogurt
- 1 garlic clove, minced
- 1 lemon, juiced
- 2 tbsp fresh dill, chopped
- 2 tbsp fresh parsley, chopped
- Salt and pepper to taste
- 4 whole-grain pita breads

Instructions:

1. Preheat your oven to 375°F (190°C).
2. In a medium bowl, mix together the Greek-style yogurt, minced garlic, lemon juice, chopped dill, and chopped parsley.
3. Season with salt and pepper to taste.
4. Cut the pita breads into wedges and place them in a single layer on a baking sheet.
5. Bake the pita chips for 10-12 minutes, or until crispy.
6. Serve the yogurt dip with the warm pita chips.

Baked Sweet Potato Fries with Avocado Aioli

Sweet potato fries are a delicious and healthy alternative to regular fries, and they are easy to make at home. This recipe takes the fries to the next level by serving them with a creamy and flavorful avocado aioli.

Ingredients:

- 2 large sweet potatoes, cut into fries

- 2 tbsp olive oil
- 1 tsp garlic powder
- 1 tsp smoked paprika
- Salt and pepper to taste

For the Avocado Aioli:

- 1 ripe avocado, peeled and pitted
- 1 garlic clove, minced
- 2 tbsp plain Greek-style yogurt
- 1 tbsp lime juice
- Salt and pepper to taste

Instructions:

1. Preheat your oven to 400°F (200°C).
2. Cut the sweet potatoes into fries and toss them in a large bowl with the olive oil, garlic powder, smoked paprika, salt, and pepper.
3. Spread the sweet potato fries in a single layer on a baking sheet and bake for 20-25 minutes, or until crispy.

4. While the sweet potatoes are baking, make the avocado aioli. In a small bowl, mash the avocado with a fork and add the minced garlic, Greek-style yogurt, lime juice, salt, and pepper. Mix well.

5. Serve the sweet potato fries with the avocado aioli.

Mini Caprese Skewers

These mini caprese skewers are the perfect appetizer for any occasion. They are easy to make and are a great way to incorporate fresh vegetables into your diet.

Ingredients:

- 1 pint cherry tomatoes
- 1 package mini fresh mozzarella balls
- Fresh basil leaves
- Balsamic glaze

Instructions:

1. Thread one cherry tomato, one mini fresh mozzarella ball, and one small basil leaf onto each skewer.

2. Arrange the skewers on a serving platter.

3. Drizzle the skewers with balsamic glaze.

4. Serve and enjoy!

Beet Hummus with Crudité

This vibrant and flavorful beet hummus is a great way to incorporate more vegetables into your diet. Serve it with a variety of fresh crudité for a healthy and satisfying snack.

Ingredients:

- 2 medium beets, peeled and chopped
- 1 can chickpeas, drained and rinsed
- 1 garlic clove, minced
- 1 lemon, juiced
- 2 tbsp tahini
- Salt and pepper to taste
- Assorted vegetables for dipping (carrots, celery, bell peppers, etc.)

Instructions:

1. Preheat your oven to 375°F (190°C).
2. Roast the chopped beets in the oven for 30-35 minutes, or until tender.
3. In a food processor, combine the roasted beets, chickpeas, minced garlic, lemon juice, tahini, salt, and pepper.
4. Pulse the mixture until smooth and creamy.
5. Serve the beet hummus with a variety of fresh crudité for dipping.

Cauliflower Buffalo Bites

These cauliflower buffalo bites are a healthy and delicious alternative to traditional buffalo wings. Serve them with a creamy ranch dip for the ultimate snack.

Ingredients:

- 1 head cauliflower, cut into florets
- 1/2 cup whole-wheat flour
- 1/2 cup water

- 1 tsp garlic powder
- 1/4 tsp salt
- 1/4 cup hot sauce
- 1 tbsp melted butter
- For the Ranch Dip:
- 1/2 cup plain Greek-style yogurt
- 1/2 tsp garlic powder
- 1/2 tsp dried dill

Instructions:

1. Preheat your oven to 450°F (230°C).
2. In a large bowl, whisk together the whole-wheat flour, water, garlic powder, and salt until smooth.
3. Add the cauliflower florets to the bowl and toss to coat evenly with the batter.
4. Arrange the coated cauliflower florets on a baking sheet lined with parchment paper and bake for 15-20 minutes, or until golden brown.
5. In a small bowl, whisk together the hot sauce and melted butter.

6. Toss the baked cauliflower florets in the hot sauce mixture until coated.

7. To make the ranch dip, mix together the Greek-style yogurt, garlic powder, and dried dill in a small bowl.

8. Serve the cauliflower buffalo bites with the ranch dip on the side.

Shrimp Cocktail with Avocado Salsa

This shrimp cocktail with avocado salsa is a fresh and flavorful appetizer that is perfect for any occasion. The tangy and zesty avocado salsa complements the succulent shrimp perfectly.

Ingredients:

- 1 lb cooked shrimp, peeled and deveined
- 1 large avocado, peeled and diced
- 1 small red onion, finely chopped
- 1 small jalapeño pepper, seeded and minced
- 2 tbsp chopped fresh cilantro
- 2 tbsp lime juice
- Salt and pepper to taste

Instructions:

1. In a large bowl, combine the cooked shrimp, diced avocado, finely chopped red onion, minced jalapeño pepper, chopped fresh cilantro, lime juice, salt, and pepper.
2. Toss the mixture gently until well combined.
3. Spoon the shrimp cocktail into glasses or bowls.
4. Serve and enjoy!

Cucumber and Hummus Bites

These cucumber and hummus bites are a quick and easy appetizer that is perfect for any occasion. They are light, refreshing, and packed with flavor.

Ingredients:

- 1 large cucumber, sliced into rounds
- 1/2 cup hummus
- 1/4 cup chopped fresh parsley

Instructions:

1. Spread a dollop of hummus onto each cucumber round.
2. Sprinkle the chopped fresh parsley on top of the hummus.
3. Serve and enjoy!

Roasted Red Pepper and Feta Dip

This roasted red pepper and feta dip is a delicious and flavorful appetizer that is perfect for parties or gatherings. Serve it with pita chips or fresh vegetables for dipping.

Ingredients:

- 1 jar (12 oz) roasted red peppers, drained and chopped
- 1/2 cup crumbled feta cheese
- 1/4 cup chopped fresh parsley
- 1 garlic clove, minced
- 1 tbsp lemon juice
- 1 tbsp olive oil

- Salt and pepper to taste

Instructions:

1. In a food processor, combine the chopped roasted red peppers, crumbled feta cheese, chopped fresh parsley, minced garlic, lemon juice, olive oil, salt, and pepper.
2. Pulse the mixture until smooth and creamy.
3. Transfer the dip to a serving bowl.
4. Serve the roasted red pepper and feta dip with pita chips or fresh vegetables for dipping.

Snacks and appetizers are an essential part of any meal or gathering, and with these ten new recipes, you can add some variety to your snack game. From savory to sweet, there's something for everyone in this chapter. Whether you're hosting a party or just looking for a quick and healthy snack, these recipes are sure to please. So go ahead and give them a try!

Chapter 5: PCOS Diet Desserts Recipes

Desserts are often seen as the ultimate indulgence, but that doesn't mean they have to be unhealthy. In fact, there are plenty of ways to enjoy sweet treats while still sticking to a healthy diet. This chapter features 10 delicious dessert recipes that are perfect for anyone with a sweet tooth.

Chocolate Avocado Mousse

Ingredients:

- 2 ripe avocados
- 1/2 cup unsweetened cocoa powder
- 1/4 cup maple syrup
- 1/4 cup almond milk
- 1 tsp vanilla extract
- Pinch of salt

Instructions:

1. Cut the avocados in half and remove the pits.
2. Scoop the avocado flesh into a food processor or blender.
3. Add the cocoa powder, maple syrup, almond milk, vanilla extract, and salt to the food processor.
4. Blend until smooth and creamy, scraping down the sides as needed.
5. Transfer the mousse to a bowl or individual serving dishes.
6. Chill in the refrigerator for at least 30 minutes before serving.

Berry and Yogurt Parfait

Ingredients:

- 1 cup plain Greek yogurt
- 1/2 cup mixed berries (such as strawberries, blueberries, and raspberries)
- 1/4 cup granola
- 1 tbsp honey

Instructions:

1. In a small bowl, mix together the Greek yogurt and honey.
2. In a separate bowl, mix together the mixed berries.
3. Layer the yogurt mixture, berries, and granola in a glass or jar.
4. Repeat the layering until all ingredients are used up.
5. Chill in the refrigerator for at least 30 minutes before serving.

Almond Flour Chocolate Chip Cookies

Ingredients:

- 2 cups almond flour
- 1/4 cup coconut oil, melted
- 1/4 cup maple syrup
- 1 tsp vanilla extract
- 1/2 tsp baking soda
- 1/4 tsp salt
- 1/2 cup dark chocolate chips

Instructions:

1. Preheat the oven to 350°F.
2. In a large bowl, mix together the almond flour, melted coconut oil, maple syrup, vanilla extract, baking soda, and salt.
3. Fold in the dark chocolate chips.
4. Roll the dough into balls and flatten slightly on a baking sheet lined with parchment paper.
5. Bake for 10-12 minutes, or until lightly golden brown.
6. Allow to cool for a few minutes before serving.

Baked Apples with Cinnamon and Walnuts

Ingredients:

- 4 apples, cored and halved
- 1/4 cup chopped walnuts
- 2 tbsp maple syrup
- 1 tsp cinnamon
- 1/4 tsp nutmeg

- Pinch of salt

Instructions:

1. Preheat the oven to 375°F.
2. In a small bowl, mix together the chopped walnuts, maple syrup, cinnamon, nutmeg, and salt.
3. Place the apple halves on a baking sheet lined with parchment paper.
4. Spoon the walnut mixture onto each apple half.
5. Bake for 20-25 minutes, or until the apples are tender and the topping is lightly golden brown.
6. Serve warm.

Low-carb Cheesecake with Berry Compote

Ingredients:

For the crust:

- 1 cup almond flour
- 1/4 cup coconut oil, melted
- 1 tbsp maple syrup

- Pinch of salt

For the cheesecake filling:

- 16 oz cream cheese, softened
- 1/2 cup Greek yogurt
- 1/2 cup erythritol
- 2 tsp vanilla extract
- 2 large eggs

For the berry compote:

- 1 cup mixed berries (such as strawberries, blueberries, and raspberries)
- 2 tbsp water
- 1 tbsp erythritol
- 1 tsp lemon juice

Instructions:

1. Preheat the oven to 325°F.

2. In a medium bowl, mix together the almond flour, melted coconut oil, maple syrup, and salt for the crust.

3. Press the crust mixture into the bottom of a 9-inch springform pan.

4. In a large bowl, beat together the softened cream cheese, Greek yogurt, erythritol, and vanilla extract for the cheesecake filling until smooth.

5. Add the eggs one at a time, beating until just combined.

6. Pour the cheesecake filling into the prepared crust and smooth out the top.

7. Bake for 45-50 minutes, or until the cheesecake is set but still slightly jiggly in the center.

8. Allow the cheesecake to cool to room temperature before chilling in the refrigerator for at least 2 hours.

9. In a small saucepan, combine the mixed berries, water, erythritol, and lemon juice for the berry compote.

10. Bring the mixture to a simmer over medium heat, stirring occasionally, until the berries have broken down and the mixture has thickened slightly.

11. Serve the cheesecake with the berry compote spooned over the top.

Chocolate Banana Chia Pudding

Ingredients:

- 1 ripe banana
- 1/2 cup unsweetened almond milk
- 2 tbsp chia seeds
- 1 tbsp unsweetened cocoa powder
- 1 tbsp maple syrup
- Pinch of salt

Instructions:

1. Mash the ripe banana in a small bowl.
2. In a separate bowl, whisk together the almond milk, chia seeds, cocoa powder, maple syrup, and salt.
3. Add the mashed banana to the almond milk mixture and stir until well combined.
4. Pour the mixture into a jar or individual serving dishes.

5. Chill in the refrigerator for at least 2 hours, or until
    set.

Lemon Blueberry Bars

Ingredients:

For the crust:

- 1 1/2 cups almond flour
- 1/4 cup coconut oil, melted
- 2 tbsp maple syrup
- 1/2 tsp vanilla extract
- Pinch of salt

For the filling:

- 3 eggs
- 3/4 cup erythritol
- 1/2 cup lemon juice
- 1/4 cup almond flour
- 1 tsp baking powder
- 1 cup fresh blueberries

Instructions:

1. Preheat the oven to 350°F.
2. In a medium bowl, mix together the almond flour, melted coconut oil, maple syrup, vanilla extract, and salt for the crust.
3. Press the crust mixture into the bottom of a 9-inch square baking dish lined with parchment paper.
4. In a large bowl, whisk together the eggs, erythritol, and lemon juice for the filling.
5. Add the almond flour and baking powder and whisk until well combined.
6. Fold in the fresh blueberries.
7. Pour the filling mixture over the prepared crust.
8. Bake for 25-30 minutes, or until the filling is set and the edges are lightly golden brown.
9. Allow to cool to room temperature before slicing and serving.

Coconut Lime Energy Balls

Ingredients:

- 1 cup unsweetened shredded coconut
- 1/2 cup raw cashews
- 1/4 cup almond flour
- 2 tbsp chia seeds
- 2 tbsp coconut oil, melted
- Zest and juice of 1 lime
- 1 tbsp honey
- Pinch of salt

Instructions:

1. In a food processor, pulse the unsweetened shredded coconut, raw cashews, almond flour, and chia seeds until the mixture is finely ground.
2. Add the melted coconut oil, lime zest and juice, honey, and salt to the food processor and pulse until the mixture comes together into a sticky dough.
3. Roll the dough into tablespoon-sized balls.

4. Place the balls on a lined baking sheet and refrigerate
   for at least 30 minutes, or until firm.

5. Store the energy balls in an airtight container in the
   refrigerator for up to a week.

Cinnamon Apple Crumble

Ingredients:

For the filling:

- 4 medium apples, peeled and chopped
- 1 tbsp lemon juice
- 1/4 cup erythritol
- 2 tsp ground cinnamon
- 1/4 tsp ground nutmeg

For the crumble:

- 1 cup almond flour
- 1/4 cup coconut oil, melted
- 2 tbsp erythritol
- 1 tsp ground cinnamon
- Pinch of salt

Instructions:

1. Preheat the oven to 350°F.
2. In a large bowl, toss the chopped apples with the lemon juice, erythritol, cinnamon, and nutmeg for the filling.
3. Transfer the apple mixture to an 8-inch square baking dish.
4. In a separate bowl, mix together the almond flour, melted coconut oil, erythritol, cinnamon, and salt for the crumble.
5. Sprinkle the crumble mixture evenly over the top of the apple mixture.
6. Bake for 30-35 minutes, or until the top is golden brown and the apples are tender.
7. Allow to cool for a few minutes before serving.

Pumpkin Pie Cheesecake Bars

Ingredients:

For the crust:

- 1 1/2 cups almond flour

- 1/4 cup coconut oil, melted
- 2 tbsp maple syrup
- Pinch of salt

For the cheesecake filling:

- 8 oz cream cheese, softened
- 1/2 cup pumpkin puree
- 1/2 cup erythritol
- 2 tsp vanilla extract
- 2 large eggs

For the pumpkin pie layer:

- 1 cup pumpkin puree
- 1/4 cup coconut milk
- 1/4 cup erythritol
- 2 tsp pumpkin pie spice
- 1 large egg

Instructions:

1. Preheat the oven to 350°F.

2. In a medium bowl, mix together the almond flour, melted coconut oil, maple syrup, and salt for the crust.

3. Press the crust mixture into the bottom of a 9-inch square baking dish lined with parchment paper.

4. In a large bowl, beat together the softened cream cheese, pumpkin puree, erythritol, and vanilla extract for the cheesecake filling until smooth.

5. Add the eggs one at a time, beating until just combined.

6. Pour the cheesecake filling over the crust and smooth out the top.

7. In a separate bowl, whisk together the pumpkin puree, coconut milk, erythritol, pumpkin pie spice, and egg for the pumpkin pie layer.

8. Pour the pumpkin pie mixture over the cheesecake layer.

9. Bake for 45-50 minutes, or until the pumpkin pie layer is set and the cheesecake layer is slightly jiggly in the center.

10. Allow the bars to cool to room temperature, then transfer them to the refrigerator to chill for at least 2 hours.

the dessert recipes in this chapter offer a variety of options for those with PCOS who are looking to satisfy their sweet tooth without compromising their health. From fruity sorbets to creamy cheesecake bars, there is something for everyone in this collection of recipes. By using alternative sweeteners and flours, as well as incorporating nutrient-rich ingredients like nuts and fruits, these desserts not only taste delicious but can also support a PCOS-friendly diet. We hope you enjoy trying out these recipes and discovering new ways to indulge in dessert while maintaining a healthy lifestyle.

Chapter 6: PCOS Diet Beverages Recipes

Beverages are an important part of our daily lives. Whether we're starting our day with a cup of coffee or tea, or unwinding after a long day with a glass of wine, beverages play a significant role in our routines. For those with PCOS, choosing the right beverages can be especially important for managing symptoms and maintaining overall health. In this chapter, we'll explore a variety of PCOS-friendly beverages that are both delicious and nutritious.

Strawberry and Mint Infused Water

Ingredients:

- 1 cup fresh strawberries, sliced
- 1/4 cup fresh mint leaves
- 1 lemon, sliced
- 8 cups of water

Instructions:

1. In a large pitcher, add the sliced strawberries, mint leaves, and lemon slices.
2. Fill the pitcher with 8 cups of water.
3. Stir the ingredients to combine.
4. Refrigerate the pitcher for at least 2 hours before serving.
5. Pour the infused water into glasses and enjoy!

Iced Matcha Latte with Almond Milk

Ingredients:

- 1 tbsp matcha powder
- 1 tbsp honey
- 1/2 cup hot water
- 1 cup almond milk
- Ice

Instructions:

1. In a small bowl, whisk together the matcha powder and honey with 1/2 cup of hot water until the mixture is smooth.
2. Pour the matcha mixture into a blender and add the almond milk and ice.
3. Blend the ingredients until the mixture is smooth and creamy.
4. Pour the iced matcha latte into a glass and serve.

Blueberry and Lavender Smoothie

Ingredients:

- 1 cup frozen blueberries
- 1/2 cup unsweetened almond milk
- 1/2 cup plain Greek yogurt
- 1 tsp dried lavender
- 1 tbsp honey
- Ice

Instructions:

1. In a blender, add the frozen blueberries, almond milk, Greek yogurt, dried lavender, honey, and ice.
2. Blend the ingredients until the mixture is smooth and creamy.
3. Pour the blueberry and lavender smoothie into a glass and enjoy!

Spiced Apple Cider

Ingredients:

- 4 cups apple cider
- 1 cinnamon stick
- 4 cloves
- 1 star anise
- 1/2 tsp ground ginger
- 1/4 tsp ground nutmeg

Instructions:

1. In a large pot, add the apple cider, cinnamon stick, cloves, star anise, ginger, and nutmeg.
2. Stir the ingredients to combine.
3. Heat the pot over medium-high heat until the apple cider is simmering.
4. Reduce the heat to low and let the spiced apple cider simmer for at least 10 minutes.
5. Remove the pot from the heat and strain the spiced apple cider into a pitcher.
6. Serve the spiced apple cider hot and enjoy!

Low-sugar Vanilla Chai Latte

Ingredients:

- 1 black tea bag
- 1/2 cup unsweetened almond milk
- 1/2 cup water
- 1/2 tsp vanilla extract
- 1/4 tsp ground cinnamon
- 1/4 tsp ground ginger

- 1/8 tsp ground cardamom
- 1/8 tsp ground cloves
- 1 tbsp honey

Instructions:

1. In a small pot, add the black tea bag, almond milk, water, vanilla extract, cinnamon, ginger, cardamom, and cloves.
2. Stir the ingredients to combine.
3. Heat the pot over medium-high heat until the mixture is simmering.
4. Reduce the heat to low and let the mixture simmer for 5-7 minutes.
5. Remove the pot from the heat and discard the tea bag.
6. Stir in the honey until it is fully dissolved.
7. Pour the low-sugar vanilla chai latte into a mug and enjoy!

Orange and Ginger Detox Water

Ingredients:

- 1 orange, sliced
- 1/4 cup fresh ginger, sliced
- 8 cups of water

Instructions:

1. In a large pitcher, add the sliced orange and ginger.
2. Fill the pitcher with 8 cups of water.
3. Stir the ingredients to combine.
4. Refrigerate the pitcher for at least 2 hours before serving.
5. Pour the detox water into glasses and enjoy!

Creamy Turmeric Latte

Ingredients:

- 1 cup unsweetened almond milk
- 1 tsp turmeric powder
- 1/2 tsp cinnamon powder

- 1/4 tsp ground ginger
- 1/8 tsp ground cardamom
- 1 tbsp honey
- Pinch of black pepper

Instructions:

1. In a small pot, add the almond milk, turmeric powder, cinnamon powder, ginger, and cardamom.
2. Stir the ingredients to combine.
3. Heat the pot over medium-high heat until the mixture is simmering.
4. Reduce the heat to low and let the mixture simmer for 5-7 minutes.
5. Remove the pot from the heat and stir in the honey and black pepper.
6. Pour the creamy turmeric latte into a mug and enjoy!

Beet and Berry Smoothie

Ingredients:

1. 1 cup frozen mixed berries
2. 1/2 cup cooked beets, chopped
3. 1/2 cup unsweetened almond milk
4. 1/2 cup plain Greek yogurt
5. 1 tbsp honey
6. Ice

Instructions:

1. In a blender, add the frozen mixed berries, cooked beets, almond milk, Greek yogurt, honey, and ice.
2. Blend the ingredients until the mixture is smooth and creamy.
3. Pour the beet and berry smoothie into a glass and enjoy!

Sparkling Watermelon Agua Fresca

Ingredients:

- 4 cups seedless watermelon, cubed
- 1/4 cup fresh lime juice
- 2 cups sparkling water
- Ice
- Fresh mint leaves for garnish

Instructions:

1. In a blender, add the watermelon cubes and lime juice.
2. Blend the ingredients until the mixture is smooth.
3. Pour the watermelon mixture into a pitcher.
4. Add the sparkling water and stir to combine.
5. Add ice to the pitcher to chill the beverage.
6. Serve the sparkling watermelon agua fresca in glasses with fresh mint leaves for garnish.

Vanilla and Blueberry Smoothie

Ingredients:

- 1 cup frozen blueberries
- 1/2 cup unsweetened almond milk
- 1/2 cup plain Greek yogurt
- 1/2 tsp vanilla extract
- 1 tbsp honey
- Ice

Instructions:

1. In a blender, add the frozen blueberries, almond milk, Greek yogurt, vanilla extract, honey, and ice.
2. Blend the ingredients until the mixture is smooth and creamy.
3. Pour the vanilla and blueberry smoothie into a glass and enjoy!

Beverages can be a fun and easy way to incorporate PCOS-friendly ingredients into your diet. From infused waters and smoothies to hot and cold beverages, there are a variety of options to choose from. By experimenting with different recipes and ingredients, you can find the perfect beverages to support your health and well-being.

CONCLUSION

Managing PCOS symptoms can be challenging, but making healthy lifestyle choices can make a big difference. In addition to eating a healthy diet, here are some other tips for living a healthy life with PCOS:

1. Exercise regularly: Regular exercise can help improve insulin sensitivity and manage weight. Aim for at least 30 minutes of moderate-intensity exercise most days of the week.

2. Get enough sleep: Lack of sleep can worsen PCOS symptoms and lead to weight gain. Aim for 7-9 hours of sleep each night.

3. Manage stress: Chronic stress can worsen PCOS symptoms, so finding ways to manage stress is important. Consider incorporating relaxation techniques such as yoga, meditation, or deep breathing into your routine.

4. Work with a healthcare professional: If you have PCOS, it's important to work with a healthcare

professional who can help you manage your symptoms. They may recommend medications, such as birth control pills or metformin, to help regulate hormones and improve insulin sensitivity.

5. Stay positive: Managing PCOS can be challenging, but staying positive and focusing on small steps can make a big difference. Celebrate your successes and don't get discouraged by setbacks.

6. Connect with others: Connecting with others who have PCOS can be a great source of support and motivation. Consider joining a support group or connecting with others online.